The Black Hair Manual

A Pocket Guide for Choosing Your Best Hair Products

AUTHOR BREANNA RUTTER

TABLE OF CONTENTS

Introduction To The Black Hair Manual

INTRODUCTION TO
THE BLACK HAIR MANUAL

"The Black Hair Manual is a little pocket guide that will help you to select your perfect hair products. A trip to your local beauty supply store or even an experience at a seminar or beauty event may heighten the confusion of knowing if a product is truly best for keeping black hair healthy. Working with black hair alone may be very easy or difficult, depending on your practices and knowledge, while also trying to understand what products are best for your hair can be pretty challenging. There are wide selections of hair products to choose from varying in all shapes, sizes, and promises and because of this, it's so easy to be tricked and fooled into constantly buying different hair products that do nothing for your hair. In this manual, I promise to help guide you to your best hair products by informing you on how to go about finding them according to their ingredients and by helping you to know how to use every product properly for your hair. And also, if it so applies, this will serve as an encouragement to every product junkie alive!

Make sure to always keep this in your purse, backpack or pocket to always be ready to help you navigate through the beauty supply store, a beauty event you may attend, or an on the whim decision to try a new product that may have caught your eye.

Please enjoy this informative read and have fun experiencing different hair products the world has to offer for you."

-Sincerely Breanna

1 THE PERFECT SHAMPOO

When shampooing black hair understand that a little shampoo goes a long way! In fact, black hair does not have to be shampooed as often as other hair types and because of this, there is the added pressure to finding the perfect shampoo that will not strip your hair of vital moisture. Commercial shampoos are usually filled with very stripping cleansing agents that often leave black hair dryer after shampoo washing your hair. Additionally, keep in mind that for the majority, it is best to detangle natural hair when it is wet and slippery and it is best to detangle relaxed hair when it is dry. As you learn to work with your hair, doing the very opposite may be best for your unique head of hair.

A good guide for knowing how often to shampoo wash black hair is at least once a week or once every two weeks. This will vary depending on the frequency of your hair product usage and the condition of your scalp and hair. You can of course only shampoo wash according to your unique needs (which would be best) by paying attention to notice buildup of hair products or dead skin, odor, or an itchy scalp. Any or all of the above are good indicators that it would be a good time to shampoo wash your hair.

I will walk you step by step through how to shampoo wash your hair properly and then, I will give you an ingredient list to guide you to choosing the best shampoo for your hair!

Natural Hair Shampoo Regimen	Relaxed Hair Shampoo Regimen
Step 1: Apply a rinse out conditioner to your hair and wait at least 5 minutes until your hair has softened.	Step1: Dry detangle in manageable sections from the tips to the roots with a seamless wide tooth comb.
Step 2: Detangle in manageable sections from the tips to the roots with a seamless wide tooth comb.	Step 2: (For New Growth) Do Step 1 from the Natural Hair Shampoo Regimen. Do a final detangle.
Step 3: Two strand twist each section and braid the very ends to prevent unraveling.	Step 3: Two strand twist each section and braid the very ends to prevent unraveling.
Step 4: Rinse out all conditioner with warm water.	Step 4: Rise out all conditioner with warm water.
Step 5: Apply shampoo directly to the scalp. Massage with fingers pads to form a lather, then allow the lather to cleanse the ends. Final rinse with warm water.	Step 5: Apply shampoo directly to the scalp. Massage with fingers pads to form a lather, then allow the lather to cleanse the ends. Final rinse with warm water.
Step 6: Pat dry hair with a towel.	Step 6: Pat dry hair with a towel.

SAFE SHAMPOO INGREDIENTS	HARSH SHAMPOO INGREDIENTS
Water	
Pure Glycerin Soap	Ammonium Laurlyl Sulfate
Cocomidopropyl Betaine	Ammonium Laureth Sulfate
Cocomidopropyl	Sodium Lauryl Sulfate
Hydroxysultaine	Disodium Mono Oleamide
Lauramide Oxide	Sulfosuccinates
Lauramide Oxide	Sulfonates
Lauramide Diethanolamine	Sodium Laureth Lauryl Sulfate
Cocamide Diethanolamine (DEA)	Triethanolamine Lauryl Sulfate
Cocamide Monoethanolamine (MEA)	

2 THE PERFECT DEEP CONDITIONER

Black hair behaves best and is most healthy when it is moisturized so it's no surprise that a good use of conditioner reinforces the health of your hair. The usage of your deep conditioner product will not be done frequently but it is vital for balancing much need moisture into your hair. You will usually notice that when the seasons have changed, you may seem to experience drier hair than normal.

A good guide for knowing how often to deep condition black hair is at least every two weeks or once a month. Deep conditioning your hair will vary depending on how tight your curl pattern is and the health condition of your hair. Tighter curl patterns (like Type 4 Hair) often needs more deep conditioning treatments than a looser curl pattern (like Type 3 Hair). You can of course only deep condition according to your unique needs (which would be best) by paying attention to notice if your hair is dry or drier than normal or if your hair doesn't offer much stretch before breaking. If it's hard to tell that you are in need to deep condition your hair, don't worry about it, just wait until it's obvious to you. Any or all of the above are good indicators that it would be a good time to deep condition your hair.

I will walk you step by step through how to deep condition your hair properly and then, I will give you an ingredient list to guide you to choosing the best deep conditioner for your hair!

Deep Condition Regimen For
Relaxed Hair and Natural Hair

Step 1: Generously apply deep conditioner to each detangled section.

Saturate the ends then work product close to the roots.

Step 2: Two strand twist and braid each section again to prevent unraveling.

Step 3: Leave on hair for 30 minutes max, or as suggested by the product.

For deep penetration, sit under a hooded dryer with a plastic shower cap for 10-15 minutes.

Step 4: Allow the hair to cool to touch and then rinse with warm water.

Step 5: Final rinse with the coolest water you can stand to close your cuticles for smooth hair.

Step 6: Pat dry hair with a towel.

SAFE DEEP CONDITIONER INGREDIENTS	HARSH DEEP CONDITIONER INGREDIENTS
Water	
Olive Oil	
Coconut Oil	
Jojoba Oil	
Avocado Oil	Petroleum
Peanut Oil	Petrolatum
Mango Oil/Butter	Lanolin
Almond Oil/Butter	Bee's Wax
Shea Oil/Butter	Dimethicone
Grapeseed Oil	Dimethiconol
Cocoa Butter	Behenoxy Dimethicone
Tea Tree Oil	Phenyl Trimethicone
Peppermint Oil	Simethicone
Castor Oil	Trimethicone
Honey	Polydimethysiloxane
Glycerin	Cyclopentasiloxane
Glycerides	Trimethylsiloxysilicates
Pathenol	PEG Modified Dimethicone
Cellulose	Dimethicone Copolyol
Polyquarternium-10	
Polyquarternium-7	
Lauric Acid (Lauryl Acid)	
Stearic Acid (Stearyl Acid)	
Linoleic Acid	
Cetyl Acid	
Behenyl Acid	
Cetyl Alcohol	

3 THE PERFECT PROTEIN TREATMENT

Protein treatments serve as a corrective treatment for black hair that lacks strength and elasticity. The effects of various hair styling practices can lead you to needing protein treatments if you are not taking preventative action against damage. Too much moisture, application of heat or over manipulation can make your hair limp and lifeless. If limp and lifeless describes the state of your hair, you are in serious need of a protein treatment!

A good guide for knowing how often to do a protein treatment on black hair will differ depending on if you have natural hair or relaxed hair. First, let's understand when to protein treat natural hair.

Natural hair will go through a protein treatment when you notice that it does not offer much "snap back." Natural hair needs a protein treatment when it looks and feels limp and lifeless and this is most noticeable directly after shampoo washing your hair. It's easier to over process natural hair with protein than relaxed hair so never protein treat natural hair on a schedule. Rather treat the hair when needed.

Relaxed hair should receive a protein treatment at least a week after your last relaxer treatment and the same applies to color treated hair. In order from an intense, to moderate, to light protein treatment you want to look for ingredients in order of; hydrolyzed protein, partially hydrolyzed protein, and proteins in food (like eggs and yogurt) in your treatment for desired results.

I will walk you step by step through how to protein treat your hair properly and then, I will give you an ingredient list to guide you to choosing the best protein treatment for your hair!

Natural Hair Protein Treatment Regimen	Relaxed Hair Protein Treatment Regimen
Step 1: Coat each detangled section of your hair with your protein treatment. Saturate the ends then work product close to the roots.	Step1: (Touched Up Roots) Do Step 1 from the Natural Hair Protein Treatment Regimen. Also apply to relaxed hair if applicable.
Step 2: Two strand twist and braid each section again to prevent unraveling.	Step 2: Two strand twist and braid each section again to prevent unraveling.
Step 3: Leave on hair as suggested by the product. For deep penetration, sit under a hooded dryer with a plastic shower cap for 10-15 minutes.	Step 3: Leave on hair as suggested by the product. For deep penetration, sit under a hooded dryer with a plastic shower cap for 10-15 minutes.
Step 4: Thoroughly rinse hair with warm water. Final rinse with the coolest water you can stand to close your cuticles for smooth hair.	Step 4: Thoroughly rinse hair with warm water. Final rinse with the coolest water you can stand to close your cuticles for smooth hair.
Step 6: Pat dry hair with a towel.	Step 6: Pat dry hair with a towel.

SAFE PROTEIN TREATMENT INGREDIENTS	HARSH PROTEIN TREATMENT INGREDIENTS
Water Partially Hydrolyzed Protein Hydrolyzed Protein Hydrolyzed Wheat Protein Wheat Protein Hydrolyzed Soy Protein Soy Protein Amino Acids Milk Protein Cholesterol Collagen Pathenol Keratin Animal Proteins like egg and Greek yogurt (for homemade protein treatments)	Petroleum Petrolatum Lanolin Bee's Wax Dimethicone Dimethiconol Behenoxy Dimethicone Phenyl Trimethicone Simethicone Trimethicone Polydimethysiloxane Cyclopentasiloxane Trimethylsiloxysilicates PEG Modified Dimethicone Dimethicone Copolyol Ammonium Laurlyl Sulfate Ammonium Laureth Sulfate Sodium Lauryl Sulfate Sulfonates Disodium Mono Oleamide Sulfosuccinates Sodium Laureth Lauryl Sulfate Triethanolamine Lauryl Sulfate

4 THE PERFECT RINSE OUT/ DETANGLING CONDITIONER

No matter if your hair is color treated, heat trained, natural, or chemically relaxed, black hair always needs a steady supply of moisture. Healthy black hair is kept moisturized to prevent it from becoming chronically dry and the key factor to most hair care regimens is an incorporation of co-washing. Co-wash means to wash your hair with conditioner alone and this is a great way to re-moisturize your hair when you are noticing that your hair is becoming a little bit dry. Use inexpensive water based moisturizing product to serve as your co-wash conditioner and your detangling conditioner because this product is usually used frequently and in large quantities.

A good guide for knowing how often to co wash black hair is at least twice a week or weekly. The frequency of your co-washes will depend on how well your hair can retain moisture. Tighter curl patterns (like Type 4 Hair) often need more moisturizing care than a looser curl pattern (like Type 3 Hair). You can of course only co-wash according to your unique needs (which would be best) by paying attention to notice if your hair is becoming dry or is feeling drier than normal. Dry hair is a good indicator that it would be a good time to co-wash your hair.

I will walk you step by step through how to co-wash your hair properly and then, I will give you an ingredient list to guide you to choosing the best co-wash conditioner/detangling conditioner for your hair!

Natural Hair Co-wash/Detangling Regimen	Relaxed Hair Co-wash/Detangling Regimen
Step 1: Generously apply the rinse out conditioner to your hair and wait at least 5 minutes until your hair has softened.	Step1: Dry detangle in manageable sections from the tips to the roots with a seamless wide tooth comb.
Step 2: Detangle in manageable sections from the tips to the roots with a seamless wide tooth comb.	Step 2: (For New Growth) Do Step 1 from the Natural Hair Co-wash/Detangling Regimen. Do a final detangle.
Step 3: Two strand twist each section and braid the very ends to prevent unraveling.	Step 3: Two strand twist each section and braid the very ends to prevent unraveling.
Step 4: Rinse out all conditioner with warm water. Final rinse with the coolest water you can stand to close your cuticles for smooth hair.	Step 4: Rinse out all conditioner with warm water. Final rinse with the coolest water you can stand to close your cuticles for smooth hair.
Step 6: Pat dry hair with a towel.	Step 6: Pat dry hair with a towel.

SAFE RINSE OUT/DETANGLING CONDITIONER INGREDIENTS	HARSH RINSE OUT/DETANGLING CONDITIONER INGREDIENTS
Water	
Olive Oil	
Coconut Oil	
Jojoba Oil	
Avocado Oil	Petroleum
Peanut Oil	Petrolatum
Mango Oil/Butter	Lanolin
Almond Oil/Butter	Bee's Wax
Shea Oil/Butter	Dimethicone
Grapeseed Oil	Dimethiconol
Cocoa Butter	Behenoxy Dimethicone
Tea Tree Oil	Phenyl Trimethicone
Peppermint Oil	Simethicone
Castor Oil	Trimethicone
Honey	Polydimethysiloxane
Glycerin	Cyclopentasiloxane
Glycerides	Trimethylsiloxysilicates
Pathenol	PEG Modified Dimethicone
Cellulose	Dimethicone Copolyol
Polyquarternium-10	
Polyquarternium-7	
Lauric Acid (Lauryl Acid)	
Stearic Acid (Stearyl Acid)	
Linoleic Acid	
Cetyl Acid	
Behenyl Acid	
Cetyl Alchohol	

5 THE PERFECT LEAVE IN MOISTURIZER

Your perfect leave in moisturizer will vary from person to person, even from someone with similar hair to yours because every head of hair has different moisturizing needs and each individual has unique preferences. It's also very important how a product makes your hair feel and what you prefer for consistency and fragrance. Everything has to be aligned before you adopt the perfect leave in moisturizing product or it isn't best for you because what if the product has the perfect consistency, gives you incredible moisture, but you can't stand the way that it smells?

A good guide for knowing how often to apply a leave in moisturizer for black hair is bi-weekly or weekly. The frequency of applying a leave in moisturizer to your hair will vary depending on how tight your curl pattern is and how well your hair can retain moisture. Tighter curl patterns (like Type 4 Hair) often need more moisturizing attention than a looser curl pattern (like Type 3 Hair). With this product, you have to experiment to find out when applying it to your hair is best. Some prefer applying on damp, wet, or dry hair. Also, if your hair tends to feel dry, try applying your leave in moisturizer with the LOC method.

LOC Method: layering products for moisture in the order of; Liquid (leave in moisturizer or water), Oil, Cream (thick consistency moisturizer/sealant like a hair butter).

I will walk you step by step through how to moisturize your hair properly and then, I will give you an ingredient list to guide you to choosing the best leave in moisturizer for your hair!

Leave In Moisturizer Regimen For
Relaxed Hair and Natural Hair

Step 1: Coat leave in moisturizer section by section on detangled hair.

Step 2: For increased moisture (if you struggle with dry hair) incorporate the LOC Method according to your preference.

Step 3: Proceed to style working on one section at a time. If you like to style dried hair, allow hair to air dry or blow dry (according to your preference).

SAFE RINSE LEAVE IN MOISTURIZER INGREDIENTS	HARSH LEAVE IN MOISTURIZER INGREDIENTS
Water	
Olive Oil	
Coconut Oil	
Jojoba Oil	
Avocado Oil	Petroleum
Peanut Oil	Petrolatum
Mango Oil/Butter	Lanolin
Almond Oil/Butter	Bee's Wax
Shea Oil/Butter	Dimethicone
Grapeseed Oil	Dimethiconol
Cocoa Butter	Behenoxy Dimethicone
Tea Tree Oil	Phenyl Trimethicone
Peppermint Oil	Simethicone
Castor Oil	Trimethicone
Honey	Polydimethysiloxane
Glycerin	Cyclopentasiloxane
Glycerides	Trimethylsiloxysilicates
Pathenol	PEG Modified Dimethicone
Cellulose	Dimethicone Copolyol
Polyquarternium-10	
Polyquarternium-7	
Lauric Acid (Lauryl Acid)	
Stearic Acid (Stearyl Acid)	
Linoleic Acid	
Cetyl Acid	
Behenyl Acid	
Cetyl Alchohol	

6 THE PERFECT OIL SEALANTS

Your choice of oil sealant will prevent your moisturizing practices from being a waste of time and effort. Throughout this pocket guide, there has been an extreme emphasis placed on keeping your black hair moisturized because healthy black hair is synonymous with moisturized hair. The purpose of using oil as a sealant is to slow down the rate of water evaporation from your hair. There is no such thing as a permanent sealant that will keep your hair moisturized forever because a sealant like that will most likely damage your hair, prevent you from effectively using heat, and make chemical treatments like coloring and relaxing ineffective.

A good guide for knowing how often to use an oil sealant for black hair is before or after applying your leave in moisturizer. If you have adopted the LOC Method, sealing your hair with oil will come before your creamy leave in moisturizer. Depending on the porosity of your hair, you may prefer lighter oils like Coconut oil or heavier oils/butters like Grapeseed oil or Shea Butter. For the majority, tighter curl patterns (like Type 4 Hair) lean more towards heavier oils/butters and looser curl patterns (like Type 3 Hair), lean more towards lighter oils. If your hair has a tendency to have a constant dryness, try thicker consistency (heavier) oils/butters and if you don't have much difficulty maintaining moisturized hair, try thinner consistency (lighter) oils.

I will walk you step by step through how to seal your hair properly and then, I will give you an ingredient list to guide you to choosing your best oil/ hair butter product for hair!

Oil Sealing Regimen For
Relaxed Hair and Natural Hair

Step 1: (Without the LOC Method)

Lightly coat fingers with your oil/butter or choice and lubricate damp hair in manageable sections at a time.

Preferably after applying your leave in moisturizer.

Step 2: (With the LOC Method)

Lightly coat fingers with your oil/butter or choice and lubricate manageable sections at a time BEFORE applying your leave in conditioner (moisturizer).

Step 3: Proceed to style working on one section at a time. If you like to style dried hair, allow hair to air dry or blow dry (according to your preference).

SAFE OIL SEALANT INGREDIENTS	HARSH OILS SEALANT INGREDIENTS
Plant/Seed Oils; Watermelon Seed Oil Alma Oil Argan Oil Olive Oil Coconut Oil Jojoba Oil Avocado Oil Peanut Oil Mango Oil/Butter Almond Oil/Butter Shea Oil/Butter Grapeseed Oil Cocoa Butter Castor Oil Honey Cetyl Alchohol Essential Oils; Tea Tree Oil Peppermint Oil	Petroleum Petrolatum Lanolin Bee's Wax Dimethicone Dimethiconol Behenoxy Dimethicone Phenyl Trimethicone Simethicone Trimethicone Polydimethysiloxane Cyclopentasiloxane Trimethylsiloxysilicates PEG Modified Dimethicone Dimethicone Copolyol

7 THE PERFECT HAIR STYLING GEL

Hair gel is an optional product unlike your other hair care products. The previous hair products mentioned are mandatory for a healthy hair care regimen but products like gel, mousse, or holding sprays are 100% optional. Your choice of hair gel in particular, will depend on your styling needs and how well your hair gel cooperates with your hair products. For light hold, watery/loose consistency hair gels can provide just a little hold but for keeping edges held smooth and slick without reverting, a stronger hold (thicker consistency) gels would be better. Experiment with different gels because even if you favor a certain consistency, hold, and fragrance, it may leave your hair flaky and/or sticky.

A good guide for knowing when to apply hair gel to black hair is depending on your styling needs. The consistency and hold of your hair gel are not synonymous with being best for certain hair textures or curl patterns. Some gels provide light, medium, or strong holds. Some women like sculpting the look of their edges (hairline) so using a strong hold gel prevents your hair from reverting. Some like a hold on their hair because their hair may be too soft or you may just want to extend the life of a hairstyle so a stronger holding gel would be better for these situations.

Also, only apply hair gel to moisturized hair and be cautious of gels that contain protein. It's much easier to add too much protein in your hair than it is to over moisturize hair.

I will walk you step by step through how to apply gel to your hair properly and then, I will give you an ingredient list to guide you to choosing the best hair gel for your hair!

Hair Gel Regimen For
Relaxed Hair and Natural Hair

Step 1: Lightly coat fingers with your gel and lubricate manageable sections at a time.

Step 2: Proceed to style!

Step 3: (For Sculpted Edges)

Use a gel with more hold and sculpt with the pads of your fingers or a soft toothbrush (commonly used).

Step 4 (Optional):

Tie down your hair (or edges) with a silk head scarf or molding strips to prevent your hair from reverting while drying.

SAFE HAIR GEL INGREDIENTS	HARSH HAIR GEL INGREDIENTS
Water	
Carbomer	
Hydrolyzed Wheat Protein	
Aloe Vera Gel/Juice	
	Petroleum
Plant/Seed Oils;	Petrolatum
Watermelon Seed Oil	Lanolin
Alma Oil	Bee's Wax
Argan Oil	Dimethicone
Olive Oil	Dimethiconol
Coconut Oil	Behenoxy Dimethicone
Jojoba Oil	Phenyl Trimethicone
Avocado Oil	Simethicone
Peanut Oil	Trimethicone
Mango Oil/Butter	Polydimethysiloxane
Almond Oil/Butter	Cyclopentasiloxane
Shea Oil/Butter	Trimethylsiloxysilicates
Grapeseed Oil	PEG Modified Dimethicone
Cocoa Butter	Dimethicone Copolyol
Castor Oil	
Honey	
Cetyl Alchohol	
Essential Oils;	
Tea Tree Oil	
Peppermint Oil	

8 THE PERFECT HAIR CARE REGIMEN

I've explained the purpose of your hair products, how often to apply them, how to apply them, and also an ingredients list for product guidance.

It's possible that you still don't understand how to implement a regimen that will work for you because from the suggested product regimens, it can make you feel as though you have to do your hair very frequent when it's actually the opposite.

Follow the graph of the suggested weekly hair care regimen. One day you may feel the need to tweak certain parts of the hair care regimen so feel free to make changes that are necessary for you.

Now that you have been equipped with a hair care regimen, in the next section, I will provide for you a hair care regimen for keeping your hair healthy when wearing weaves and braids!

Natural Hair Care Regimen	Relaxed Hair Care Regimen
Day 1 Shampoo(mandatory) Deep Condition (optional) Moisturizer (mandatory) Oil Sealant (mandatory) Hair Gel (optional)	Day 1 Shampoo(mandatory) Deep Condition (optional) Moisturizer (mandatory) Oil Sealant (mandatory) Hair Gel (optional)
Day 2	Day 2
Day 3	Day 3
Day 4 Co-wash (optional) Moisturizer(optional) Oil Sealant (optional) Hair Gel (optional)	Day 4 Co-wash (optional) Moisturizer(optional) Oil Sealant (optional) Hair Gel (optional)
Day 5	Day 5
Day 6	Day 6
Day 7	Day 7
Week 2 Day 1 Protein Treatment (optional) Moisturizer (mandatory) Oil Sealant (mandatory) Hair Gel (optional)	Week 2 Day 1 Protein Treatment (mandatory) Moisturizer (mandatory) Oil Sealant (mandatory) Hair Gel (optional)

9 THE PERFECT REGIMEN FOR WEAVES AND BRAIDS

One of the most frequently asked hair care question is how to take care of your hair in weaves and braids. It's no surprise that this is a very common question of concern because a large percentage of black women are consumers of hair extensions. No matter if someone has natural hair or relaxed hair, it's not an uncommon thing to wear hairstyles like Sew Ins, Micro Braids, Box Braids, and Cornrow Braids for example.

Have you ever removed your braids or weaves and noticed that your hair was extremely dry or damaged and in extreme cases, begin to shed from breakage? When this happens, most people will blame their hairstylist because there hair was not in that state of condition before the stylist did their hair so blaming them is the best way to rationalize it. If you do not implement a hair care regimen when wearing weaves and braids, there is a good chance you will suffer with chronically dry hair or damaged hair with breakage.

To care for your hair underneath your install, dilute your hair products with water in separate applicator bottles for easy application. Every product has to be of a watery consistency to reach your scalp and hair effectively without leaving behind residue. This hair care regimen is suggested for at least a once a week or once every two weeks when wearing weaves and/or braids. If you exercise, implement this regimen weekly instead of once every two weeks.

The regimen is applicable for those with natural hair and relaxed hair.

The Hair Care Regimen for Weaves and Braids

Step 1: Dilute your shampoo in an applicator bottle with water until you reach a watery consistency.
Generously squirt it directly on your scalp, massage your scalp with the pads of your fingers, gently smooth the soap down your braids or weave.

Thoroughly rinse out all traces of shampoo with warm water.

Step 2: Dilute your conditioner in an applicator bottle with water until you reach a watery consistency.
Generously squirt it directly on your hair, massage your hair and scalp with the pads of your fingers, gently smooth the conditioner down your braids or weave.

Thoroughly rinse out all traces of conditioner with warm water.

Step 3: Lightly coat fingers with your oil sealant and glide your fingers across all areas of your scalp.

Step 4: Dilute your moisturizer in an applicator bottle with water until you reach a watery consistency.
Apply a light coat of moisturizer to your hair.

Step 5: Sit under a hooded dryer or bonnet dryer to dry your hair.

Step 6: At about 80% dry, apply a light coat of oil to your hair. Dry your hair thoroughly then style with more moisturizer and hair gel (optional).

AFTERWORDS

"This pocket guide was made to help you find the best products for black hair. You may have chosen to read this guide because you support my work, you were looking for the best products for your hair, or you were looking for the best products that would help out a loved one.

When I was younger, it wasn't easy finding the best hair products for my hair because I didn't know how to measure what was best for my hair. When you are not knowledged about what black hair needs, and which products can meet those needs, you will often struggle with damaged hair. In my book, The Natural Hair Bible: The 10 Commandments of Black Hair Care, I went in depth about the basic fundamentals of hair care but in this pocket guide, it was my main focus to highlight hair products, their ingredients, and proper applications.

Think about cooking for example, you can have the best ingredients imported from all parts of the world, but you don't know how to cook! And the worst part about it is that you decided to go forth with best efforts without a cook book!

This pocket guide is a resource for healthy black hair and for hair fanatics as well!

Thanks for reading, it was a pleasure of mine to write this for your knowledge and enjoyment."

Sincerely, Breanna

ADDITIONAL RESOURCES

The Official Website: www.Howtoblackhair.com
The Online Store: www.HowtoblackhairStore.com
Free Subscription Email: http://eepurl.com/FZs5b

For Additional Hair Questions
YourHairQuestions@Gmail.com

Black Hair Styling Tutorials

BlackWomenHair YouTube Channel
www.Youtube.com/BlackWomenHair

HowToBlackHair YouTube Channel
www.Youtube.com/HowToBlackHair

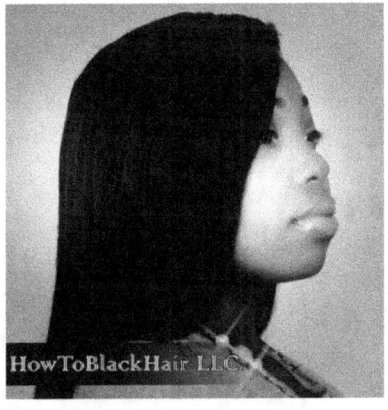

HAIR TSHIRTS + DVDS

My Creatively Designed Hair T-Shirts are Available Now!
www.Howtoblackhair.com "Click the Store Tab"

Other Designs, Sweatshirts, Phone Cases, and much more
AVAILABLE as well!

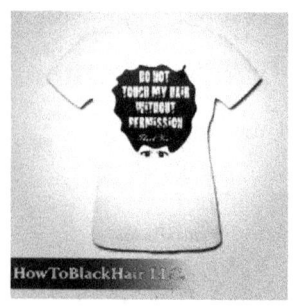

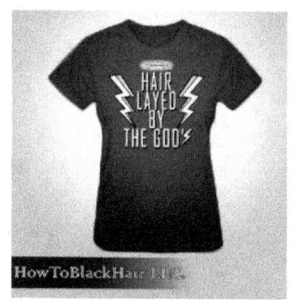

"Do Not Touch My Hair"
T-Shirt

"Hair Layed By The Gods"
T-Shirt

Over 20 Black Hair Styling DVDs
www.Howtoblackhair.com "Click the Store Tab"

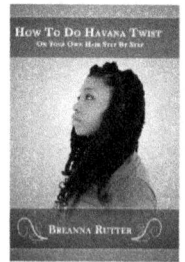

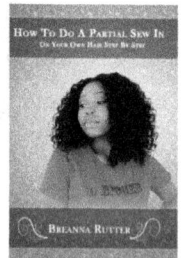

DEFINITION GUIDE

Colored Hair: *hair that has been colored*

Curl Pattern: *the look of your curls based on the LOIS or Andre Walker Hair Typing System*

Cuticles: *the scales along the outside of your hair follicle are responsible for preventing protecting the health of your hair*

Dry Detangle: *to detangle the hair while it is dry. Lubricating the hair with oil and then detangling is still dry detangling*

Elasticity: *the stretching ability of your hair.*

Hair Texture: *the feel of your hair usually falling within three different types of textures; silky, cottony and/or thready*

Lather: *to produce a frothy airy mass from your hair products*

LOC Method: *layering products for moisture in order of; Liquid (leave in moisturizer or water), Oil, Cream (thick consistency moisturizer/sealant like a hair butter)*

Natural Hair: *hair that has not received a relaxer treatment*

New Growth: *the roots of your hair that has not received a relaxer treatment*

Product Junkie: *someone who jumps from one product or another or has a large collection of hair products.*

Regimen: *the implementation of hair products and manipulation techniques used for healthy hair care*

Relaxed Hair: *hair that has received a relaxer treatment*

Retain Moisture: *the ability to keep moisturized hair even after it has dried*

Sealant: *using an oil or oil based hair product to form a temporary barrier around wet hair*

Seamless Wide Tooth Comb: *a comb with no seams to be felt within the binding teeth of the comb that will aggravate your hair and cause breakage*

Type 3 Hair: *the appearance of the curl looks more like wide spirals and not like tight coils or springs or waves*

Type 4 Hair: *the appearance of the curl looks more like tight coils and springs rather than wide spirals or waves*

INDEX

VISIT WWW.HOWTOBLACKHAIR.COM

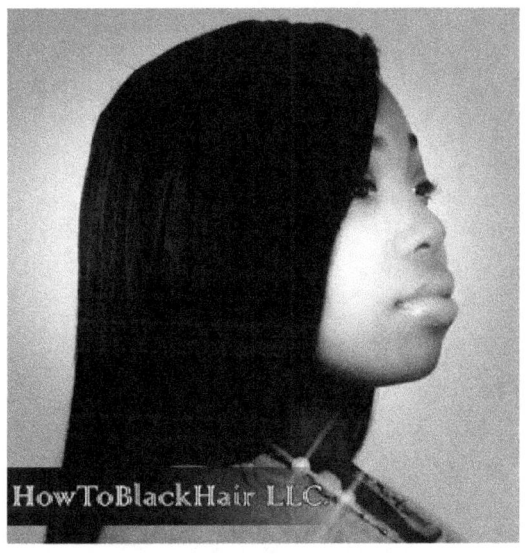

DISCLAIMER: All suggestions, techniques and advice given are for informational purposes only and should be used at your discretion and best judgment. I highly recommend conducting strand tests when trying or using new products, hair appliances and product mixes. I am not responsible or liable for adverse or undesirable affects including hair loss, hair breakage or other hair/scalp/skin/body damage as a direct or indirect result of the suggestions, tips, techniques and/or advice given.